I0415380

Coping

and

Hoping

With Infertility

By Samantha Garner

Copyright © 2019 by Samantha Garner
All rights reserved. This book or any portion thereof
may not be reproduced or used in any manner whatsoever
without the express written permission of the publisher
except for the use of brief quotations in a book review.

First Printing, 2019

ISBN 9781098761714

www.copingandhoping.com

The book is presented to provide helpful information on the subjects
discussed. This book is not meant to be used, nor should it be used, to
diagnose or treat any medical condition. For diagnosis or treatment of
any medical problem, consult your own physician. Neither the author
nor the publisher is responsible for any specific health needs that may
require medical supervision and they are not liable for any damages or
negative consequences from any treatment, action, application or
preparation, to any person reading or following the information in this
book.

For Allison,

for Becky,

and for Adam

I am writing to you from the first day of my period. It's been months...and months...years...and years. You'd think by now I'd know what to expect. That I wouldn't get my hopes up. That, damn it, I might just relax, let it happen, have faith.

Nope. I spent the morning sobbing. First in bed. Then in my husband's arms. In the shower, past when all the hot water ran out and cycled back again, which I didn't know was a thing.

I can't get pregnant. There's nothing medically wrong with me, nor with my spouse.

I can't get you pregnant. I've never been pregnant, I'm not a medical professional, and I'm not a prophet. But I've coped-as best I can.

This book is not for you innocent women, still naively believing the great reproductive myth: if you have unprotected sex you will get pregnant.

This book is for us battle-worn women, who've done the dirty, visited the doctor, peed on ovulation tests, and still, month after heart-breaking month, and still gotten a big fat negative pregnancy test. We're in it together, although sometimes it doesn't feel like it.

I still can't quite give up hope, although logic and statistics are against me. We haven't given up yet.

The reason behind this book, honestly, is because it's a tool I desperately need. I hope it will help you. It's helping me just form these words on the page. But I wanted a place of my own to record my thoughts, to keep it all straight. To observe my patterns, to record thoughts and hopes and prayers. To come to terms with the fact that I have no control in the most important decision of my life.

We Can Dream, Can't We?

I think about my baby all the time. Obsessively. It seems impossible to miss someone I've never met, but I do! It's a constant ache in my heart. I found that it helps to give my baby a name. To be clear, this is not any name you would actually put on a birth certificate. You'd be laughed out of the hospital maybe for using it. But it's a nice, gender-neutral nickname for you to use when thinking about your baby.

Some examples:
Baby
Sweetpea
Honey
Silly
Sweety
Buddy
Precious
Little One
A composite of meaningful names (Renesme anyone?-seriously, though, you can come up with cute ones; my mother is Karen and my mother-in-Law is Lynette, so mine would be Karette/Carrot; my sister's mother-in-Law is Rosie, so hers would be Kosie/Cozy)

You get it. These are not names to use, and (like a wish) it might not work if you tell others what it is.

And so, here write your baby's name, a name you can use throughout this book to refer to your wished-for baby.

_____

You Have Sex, You Get Pregnant, Right?

Somehow most of us are never taught about our bodies. Sex-ed in school's goal is to keep us from getting pregnant. I was watching a t.v. show in which the character had unprotected sex and the next day craved an apple and therefore she became convinced that she was pregnant. The next day she got her period and was relieved. Whoa. Not only is that wrong, it is impossible, and the worst part is I would never have second guessed it if I haven't had to teach myself about my own body. This conception thing takes a couple of weeks. Let's look at how our bodies work over a month. This is my simplified summary of some heavy duty biology.

Phase One: Your period. Bleeding and spotting. Need I say more?

Phase Two: Follicular Phase. Admittedly my favorite part, because I get to drink, have sex for fun, and it's the only time of the month when I'm neither in mourning nor anxious for the next month's outcome. It's the little things. Anyway, your body is prepping for ovulation.

Phase Next: Fertility Window to Ovulation. Baby making time. Your body prepares for conception by increasing hormones, making you-ahem-amorous (okay, horny), opening your cervix up (sounds hot), producing sperm-loving cervical mucus (oh yeah), and preparing your egg for release, which it does (if all goes according to plan). Have sex every night or every other night. If scheduled sex is not so fun for you, you're not alone. More on this to come. No pun intended.

Luteal Phase: The Two Week Wait. Anxiety. Every headache, cramp, change in temperature feels significant. Here's the thing, though: it will take about a week or two for your body to even register you're pregnant, if you are. You release an egg and then it just chills in your fallopian tubes for a few hours, to about a day, maybe a little over. Wow that's a small window. I mean, really we only have about a day to conceive. That being said, sperm can live for a few days, which is why people can get pregnant by having sex on days when they're not ovulating. It takes the egg, whether fertilized or not, anywhere from six days to two weeks to make it down the fallopian tube to the uterus. It takes another day or so to implant, meaning burrow its way into the uterine lining if it's fertilize. Sadly, if it's not fertilized it will just get swept out; you will not be able to see it, because it is so small. So, if your egg is fertilized, it takes a week or two to actually become pregnant. In that time your body doesn't know whether it is or not, as far as we know. If a fertilized egg implants you might have a few signs, symptoms such as cramping, headaches, back pain, spotting, breast tenderness...but all of those are also signs of your period coming so it's hard to count on them. Anyway, once it does implant your body will start making the pregnancy hormone, hCG, which is what home pregnancy tests detect when you pee on them. For every day pregnant your body will double the amount of hCG, so if you think you're pregnant but the test is negative wait a couple of days (if you can wait that long) and try again.

The big take-away from this is: the two week wait is that...a wait. Some people claim to know the second their egg is fertilized or the next day or something. No. I'm not one to dismiss hunches, so if that's what it is, then great. But you will not be craving things, feeling nauseous, gaining weight, etc. These symptoms can accompany ovulation, but wait a week or two before you read into every little thing. And once you ovulate you cannot get pregnant, so a few days before your period is not a fertile window (I'm talking to you, Lorelei Gilmore).

Charting and Ovulation Predictor Kits: The Illusion of Control

The thing about both is that they are not one-hundred percent effective and their actual efficiency is usually only apparent in retrospect.

For me, I wasted months trying to conform my body to the typical 28 day cycle, with ovulation occurring on the 14th day. It's a pretty picture, but it turns out I don't ovulate until much later in my cycle and seldom regularly, so it was not helpful. Even so, usually it happens around Day 19 of my cycle, but it's randomly happened as early as Day 10. You can't count on Day 14 being it for you.

Then I diligently tracked my ovulation according to urine based kits. Guess what? According to my basal body temperature I ovulate 3-4 days after the kit said "go."

Later, I tracked cervical mucus (sounds gross, but what're we going to do?) and basal body temperature. Okay, still not pregnant, but when I look back on my chart I feel like there's some pattern there, and I recommend it. According to most doctors cervical mucus is the best and only really sure sign of fertility.

For a clear and totally doable approach, use the spaces on the provided journal later in this book. On the next page is a brief explanation of what's what, but if you want a more in depth study read Toni Weschler's *Taking Charge of Your Fertility*. It should be required reading for every woman (and it wouldn't hurt men, either), whether you're trying to conceive or not.

The thing about this journey we call trying to conceive, I have been flummoxed by all that I didn't and don't know about my own body.

We're all willing to try anything at this point, right? So let's talk about charting. It's a pretty easy way to look at patterns in your cycle. With a little practice you can start to pick out your most fertile days and give yourself the best chance.

Cycle Day: What day in your cycle are you? Day 1 is your first day of flow.

BBT: Basal Body Temperature: Take your temperature first thing in the morning, before you even get out of bed. I use a regular digital thermometer, but there are specialized BBT ones out there, if you choose. Write it down to the tenth of a degree. To be honest, I don't bother with it during my period. Once I'm officially in the Follicular Phase I do, and in this phase you can expect lower temperatures that are generally consistent. Some exceptions might occur based on factors like illness, heavy drinking, a change in schedule, or even if you got up in the middle of the night. Some lucky few get a special cue from their bodies that they are about to ovulate with a dip in temperatures right beforehand, but this is unusual and unreliable. Once there is a large jump in temperature, this signifies ovulation; once this has happened your temperature will jump a whole degree or so. For me, my Follicular Phase temps are in the mid 97's, with a jump into the mid to upper 98's after ovulation. If you are really really really lucky you may notice a third jump after a week or so...congratulations, this might mean you're pregnant! I'm envious, but happy for you. Or it'll drop back down and we start again.

What causes the leap is a rise in progesterone after ovulation, which keeps your body from ovulating again, or, if you're pregnant, from menstruating.

I like charting. It makes me feel knowledgeable and a bit in control. That said, you can make yourself crazy with it. Every month I search for pregnancy charts on the internet and painstakingly compare my chart, interpreting every dip and rise. Chart, but try not to obsess. I know, I know: easier said than done.

Your luteal phase is from ovulation until your next period. For most people it's more than ten days long, and any less may represent a progesterone problem. The typical is twelve to fourteen days long. Luteal phases are pretty consistent from cycle to cycle so if you notice your luteal phase is a couple of days longer than normal you should take a pregnancy test. Good luck!

CM: Cervical Mucus: Sounds gross, but that's exactly what it is. It's the stuff that comes out of you. Down there. We all have a degree of discharge throughout our cycles; this is normal and healthy. We have menstruation and spotting, then a dry-ish few days with a dry kind of discharge. We get a few days of wet/sticky. And then...egg-white. That's what it's described as. This is the baby-making holy grail. It looks like raw egg white coming out of you. It stretches. It's not sticky but holds strong. If/when you see this, it's go-time. Get busy. If you don't get this, that's okay, too, because you can still conceive in the general "wet" phase. Just don't confuse it with sexual arousal, which is a different thing. Gosh it's hard to keep it all straight. Once your discharge goes away or is dry again, then you've ovulated and it's time to begin the dreaded two-week wait. A final note: if you notice a change in your CM or discharge, such as smell or color, this may be sign of a medical issue and you should seek medical attention.

CO: Cervical Opening: Your vagina is not very big. You can probably touch your cervical opening with your finger tip. Essentially what you're doing is determining how open it is, because around ovulation the opening expands. Otherwise it's closed. I think the best way to get the feel for it is...to feel for it. Start exploring in the days leading up to ovulation after a month or two of charting, once you have a sense of your personal timeline. It takes a while to start to really notice the difference. This is not as important, in my opinion, as CM, which is much more definite and noticeable. And this can feel awkward. Very.

Notes: Anything that may have impacted the other categories, such as if you were ill or traveled. You can also note symptoms, like if you get breast tenderness around ovulation or really weepy the day before your period. Just me then? Here, too, you can include unusual symptoms or side-effects of medication. For example, I was freaking out once when I started spotting mid-cycle, but because I was charting I saw it lined up with ovulation and may have been a result of some new supplements I was taking.

Or you may prefer to chart Basal Body Temperature visually on a graph, at least to start. I'll simply advise you to do an internet search for "fertility charting" or "basal body temperature chart." To provide you with one would be reinventing the wheel and perhaps copyright infringement.

Preggos Are Not the Enemy! But I Hate Those Bitches.

Not fair, but I straight up cannot be around pregnant women without fuming and/or crying. I started avoiding my cousin around the holidays, because she conceived without trying. Seriously, haven't talked to her in two years. So. How to deal, right?

Try to be happy for them. It's what you would want. They deserve it. Or at least they don't not deserve a baby. But the thing is, I can't help but compare myself. I start thinking about why I deserve to have a baby more than they do. Then, within seconds, I think to myself: "no wonder I don't have a baby. I'm so mean and judgmental." And then follows a spiraling down of why I'm the worst and why I'll never have a baby. Oh my gosh I hope that sounds crazy to you and your thoughts don't go that direction at all. Yes, drug-users, starving people, people in warzones, people who have only had sex one time, people who used a condom and pulled out and took Plan B...they get pregnant. But we're not. It does no good to compare. We're not pregnant, but they are. There's really nothing to do except try to focus on your own journey.

And you know what? Maybe, when we do have a baby, we'll appreciate it more. I know if/when I get pregnant and I'm barfing all the time due to morning sickness and my insides become my outsides during labor, when I'm exhausted from lack of sleep from a screaming infant, and when my toddler throws a fit, I'll be able to smile and thank my lucky stars that I even have a baby. I know it's not much of a bright side, but to some extent I think it's true that if you work hard for something and have to wait a long time for it, you'll value it all the more. I know plenty of parents who got knocked up right away and do nothing but complain, or after the first one is out start on making another, without taking the time to really revel in the experience. Who knows? Maybe we're the lucky ones? Of course not. But it's something. It's taking the short end of the stick. It's making the most of a bad situation.

I've also made more and closer connections to other aspiring mothers. We are a real community and nothing compares to the giant heart-hole that is infertility. Reach out to other women and hear their stories. You're not alone.

So what to do around Preggos.

Option One: Try to be happy for them. If you're close enough to them, maybe you can share in some of their joy. Throw a baby shower, go to a doctor's appointment, discuss names (but don't be too opinioned; this is, after all, their baby), buy clothes and toys, go maternity shopping. When the baby comes, babysit! The new mom will appreciate it and you'll get a small baby fix. And who knows? When it's your turn they'll be more likely to reciprocate all those things.

Option Two: Have a mature conversation with mom-to-be and other people. If you have a co-worker, friend, family member, neighbor, etc. who is expecting, explain your situation. "I'm so happy for you, but I've been trying to conceive, unsuccessfully, for x amount of time. I would really appreciate it if you minimize the baby talk around me. I won't be able to come to your baby shower, because it will make me too sad, but really I wish you all the best. Thank you for understanding."

Option Three: This is my go-to, I'll admit it. Ignore them and avoid them. Avoid places they'll be, do not engage in conversation. Employ a friend to run interference, so if you're around a Preggo they can change the subject if Preggo starts talking babies.

So You Got Your Period

This is the worst. Not only do we feel the devastation of finding out we're not pregnant, but we have hormones amplifying our feelings. The first day of my period is the worst. I wonder if there's any point to my life. If I'll ever be a mother. If I deserve to be a mother. It's dark. If ever you get so depressed that you feel suicidal, seek medical attention immediately. Call 911 or the National Suicide Prevention Hotline at 1-800-273-8255.

Feeling that way is more common than we think and help is out there. Seriously. Studies have shown anxiety, depression, anger, and grief levels among infertile women to be comparable to people diagnosed with terminal diseases.

One thing I found really helped me is keeping a list of things I love to do for me that are not baby related. Sometimes it's enough to just make the list and remind yourself that there is more to your life than trying to conceive. It's easy to lose sight of that.

Make a list and turn to it when you need something to do to pick yourself up. Try to think of 34 things you love to do, no matter how small or weird. If 34 seems like an arbitrary number to you, take heart in knowing that I chose it for a specific purpose: because that's how many fit on a page. The point I'm trying to make here is there's no right number. Think of as many as you can. If it takes you a few months to fill this list up, that's fine. If you need more, then scribble in the margins, write on a post it and stick it on top. Whatever works for you.

1. _____

2. _____

3. _____

4. _____

5. _____

6. _____

7. _____

8. _____

9. _____

10. _____

11. _____

12. _____

13. _____

14. _____

15. _____

16. _____

17. _____

18. _____

19. _____

20. _____

21. _____

22. _____

23. _____

24. _____

25. _____

26. _____

27. _____

28. _____

29. _____

30. _____

31. _____

32. _____

33. _____

34. _____

Okay, this next one is hard. Imagine the very first few minutes you hold your baby. Try to leave gender out of it, but otherwise be as realistic and specific as possible.

It's a struggle to do, even painful, but there are a few reasons to do so.

For one, sometimes picturing what you're working toward can make it all seem more worthwhile. Yes, getting your period when you're trying to conceive can feel like the end of hope, but this is why we're putting ourselves through all this.

Secondly, visualizing what you want can be a powerful force. You might consider it a sort of visual prayer or message to the universe. Either way, studies have shown a positive impact with visualizing your goals. Perhaps a small part of it is that you are focusing on the positive aspects of this journey we call having a baby, instead of the negatives. Changing your mindset, trying to be optimistic, finding joy in it...these can all help you cope with the disappointment, frustration, and sorrow.

That being said, feel free to skip this part or come back to it later.

What do you look like? _____

_____

_____

_____

Is a partner/spouse/family/friend/doula with you? Where? What are they doing?

_____

How do you feel? _____

_____

_____

_____

_____

What are the first words you say to your baby? _____

_____

_____

Describe the environment around you, including colors, music, noise: _____

_____

_____

_____

_____

If you already have a child/stepchild, how will you introduce them?

_____

_____

_____

Sex: Whether You Want To...Or Not

Sex is the most common and traditional way of getting pregnant. However, nothing can kill the mood quite like a.) scheduling sex, b.) the pressure to conceive, c.) doing it when you're not in the mood but have to, d.) getting your spouse/partner to have sex when they're not in the mood, thereby leading to e.) you getting angry/frustrated/feeling rejected and then wanting the baby-making even less.

You need to determine how much information you're going to share with your spouse/partner. Some couples chart together, go to every appointment together, and can freely discuss menstruation, ovulation, the quality of cervical mucus, and other intimate details. If you do, great!

If not, that's okay, too. Sometimes it's easier to leave men in the dark. Try to explain the basics, keeping in mind that most people haven't had the birds and the bees talk for ten to twenty years by the time they're trying to conceive, plus that talk was focused on not getting pregnant. He needs to understand that there is a small window of possibility for conception. As you chart or track your ovulation you'll have a better and better idea of when that may be. He needs to know that his services will be required the three to five days leading up to ovulation (but for goodness sake don't say it like that!). If his sperm count is low, some say to have sex every other day, otherwise try to have sex the day of, the day after, and one or two of the days before.

My husband knows my euphemisms by now. For example, "date night" means "I'm ovulating soon and you'd better be ready to have sex no matter what". The first phrase is much more pleasant to hear and takes the pressure off a little. My friend tells her spouse to "save his love for her", a coded way of saying: "don't masturbate," because (of course) we need every last swimmer.

There may be times when he is just not in the mood at all. If you can persuade him to have a beer, take a shower, go for a jog, watch "adult" videos...whatever works to get ready, then great. Go for it! But if you get in a fight about having sex it'll only make it worse for both of you. With all the work and stress we're under, it's very hard to cut him any slack. I mean, come on! All he has to do is have an orgasm! Sounds delightful, right? He may not say it, but he's bound to be feeling anxiety and stress by this point. Every so often give him a pass. Then try again tomorrow.

If you're like me, however, you're not going to often give yourself a pass. Yes, around ovulation our hormones tend to rev up our sex drives, but the stress of trying to conceive can make sex seem like a chore. For those days, I recommend you use Pre-Seed. It's a lubricant that's safe for sperm; everything else, including saliva and natural oils, inhibits motility and can even kill them.

And yet, this can be a time of great intimacy. You can let loose, because you no longer have to worry about taking a pill or using a condom. Yay! Think how much money you don't have to waste on birth control! You've also committed to your spouse/partner on a whole new level by deciding to have their baby. Now that's a lifelong commitment!

If you're wondering, no position has been definitively proven to be more effective than any other, although most experts suggest a position that allows for the deepest penetration, like plain ol' missionary, because the closer he can get to those eggs to start, the better. That is not scientifically proven, though. Some people suggest putting a pillow under your bum to use gravity to pull the sperm toward your egg and lying still for about fifteen minutes. Again, this is not scientifically proven, but it can't hurt.

This could also be a time to have fun with sex. Buy some naughty lingerie, act out a fantasy, try something new, take a little trip somewhere, go shopping together in a sex shop, sext each other...

Make notes of some things you can do on those days when one or both of you aren't quite feeling it. Sometimes even just thinking about sex itself (and not baby-making) can do the trick.

When you're not feeling it: _____

_____

_____

When he's not feeling it: _____

_____

_____

When no one's feeling it: _____

_____

_____

_____

You could fill out both, have him fill out his and you fill out yours, or swap for a sexy surprise in a month or two.

I'm So Excited!

Being a parent is going to be wonderful and the most important thing we'll ever do, unless you're Batman or something. In the spirit of remaining optimistic, of visualizing the joy of being a parent, make a list here of some of things you're most excited about when you become a parent.

1. _____

2. _____

3. _____

4. _____

5. _____

6. _____

7. _____

8. _____

9. _____

10. _____

11. _____

12. _____

14. _____

15. _____

16. _____

17. _____

18. _____

19. _____

20. _____

21. _____

22. _____

23. _____

24. _____

25. _____

I'm So Scared!

But what about some of your anxieties? That's a real part of this journey. Will my baby be happy and healthy? Will I be a good mama? Will my body be destroyed by giving birth? Oh my gosh, I could fill a second book with my fears and concerns. Get them off your chest. This is a safe space!

1. _____
2. _____
3. _____
4. _____
5. _____
6. _____
7. _____
8. _____
9. _____
10. _____
11. _____
12. _____

14. _____
15. _____
16. _____
17. _____
18. _____
19. _____
20. _____
21. _____
22. _____
23. _____
24. _____
25. _____

I Dream of Baby

And now a few others things that will both break your heart and fill you with joy to think about. Form a picture of your baby in your mind. Not just what they look like at birth, but as they grow into toddlers, children, teens, and beyond. This takes a stretch of the imagination, but if it's a challenge just think about how you and/or your spouse/partner looked at various ages.

At this point in the book, just describe your baby at about 6 months to one year.

Hair color: _____

Hair texture: _____

Eye color: _____

Skin color: _____

Smile: _____

Height: _____

Weight: _____

What will your baby call you as they learn to speak? (mom, mother, mum, mummy, mama...etc.)

_____

What will your baby call your spouse/partner?

_____

What will your baby call their grandparents? Aunts? Uncles? Siblings? Your friends?

_____

_____

_____

What lullabies will you sing to your baby?_____

_____

_____

What theme will their room be? _____

What will you do for your baby's first birthday? _____

_____

_____

What books do you want to read together? _____

_____

_____

I know how crazy, stupid, hard this part is. However, I think by picturing your baby you'll remember why it's all worth it. It's all for the chance at loving that little one.

Lifestyles of the Fertile and Pregnant

Here is some general information on making your body as baby-compatible as possible:

1. Eat healthily. This may be different for everyone, but a major study concluded that the best diet for making a baby includes: a lot of vegetables and whole grains, clean and lean protein from fish and/or plant-based sources (beans and lentils), full fat products, low to no added sugar, and little to no processed food.

2. Get regular check-ups. This means going to a general practitioner and running blood work and getting a physical. Additionally, dental hygiene is important and there have been links between infertility and dental problems. Weird, but true.

3. Maintain a healthy BMI (between 18.5 and 24.9). Calculate it by multiplying your weight in pounds by 703, then divide that by your height in inches squared, or: BMI= (pounds x 703) / (height in inches x height in inches). Or, better yet, do an internet search for BMI calculator, input your height and weight, and voila.

4. Do gentle exercise. Walking, pilates, yoga, swimming...anything that is low impact. Intense exercise can disrupt ovulation and even menstruation. Also, intense exercise can stress the body, leading to inflammation and can mess with your hormones. There are tons of free videos online that are specific exercises for fertility and pregnancy. Of course, always check with your medical professional before starting any exercise.

5. Limit caffeine intake. This one can be tough! Some say it's okay and doesn't affect fertility. One doctor told me as long as I was down to one cup of coffee by my third trimester I would be okay.

But a lot of sources indicate that there may be a relationship between them, with most experts suggesting limiting your total daily caffeine intake to 200mg, which is one small cup of coffee. I switched to one to two cups of decaf a day, plus hot teas (herbal and decaffeinated). I'll still have a cup of caff or half-caff here and there.

6. Limit or cut out alcohol. Many experts say that for women, more than one serving of alcohol a day is considered "moderate," with eight servings a week being considered "heavy." I have to admit, this is my favorite vice. I don't drink once I've ovulated just in case, but come on! It helps with cramps on my period, it relaxes me, it's a part of my social life, and-damn it-I like the way it tastes! If you've been trying for a while, though, it might be time to cut back or ditch it altogether.

7. Try organic. It can be tough and more expensive, but I rationalize that a couple of dollars difference on some food is cheaper than IVF. This one is controversial, but it certainly can't hurt. Buying food that is in season means it is much cheaper. I buy featured food that is on sale, and I buy grains, nuts, and beans in bulk. Frozen fruits and veggies are thought to be about as healthy as the fresh, if there's nothing added. Finally, shopping at farmer's markets and grocery stores that identify as organic/health food stores (such as Whole Foods, Sprouts, Wegmans, Trader Joe's, Lucky's, and perhaps some local stores) tend to have a wider variety of in season fruits and veggies at lower costs than supermarkets. This may be harder in small towns, but do what you can; some food can even be ordered online and delivered to your home. At least avoid what's known as "the dirty dozen," foods that have the most chemicals known to harm humans. It changes from time to time, so do an internet search to determine which ones you may want to switch to organic.

8. Don't smoke. Maybe this one should have been higher on the list, but we all know it's bad for us, so you have to figure it's bad for a baby. No cigarettes, no cigars, no vaping, no marijuana...and if you are around people who smoke, ask them to give you some distance or take it outside, because second-hand smoke is bad news, too.

9. No drugs that aren't prescribed. Make sure any prescriber knows you are trying to conceive and ask if they are pregnancy safe, just in case. Of course: no hard drugs. A lot of over the counter medicines can be harmful to fertility and to a developing baby.

10. Find some joy. Whatever that means to you, the happier you are and the more positive your thoughts the better you'll be. See previous lists.

11. Some chemicals, perhaps from your work or even around the house cleaners, can negatively affect fertility.

12. Get some sleep! Everyone is different, but at least seven and not more than nine is considered ideal. And experts agree: you can't make up sleep! So don't think you can run on a few per night then sleep for twelve hours on the weekend; it doesn't work like that. Keep your sleeping schedule consistent within an hour every day of the week.

13. Take a prenatal vitamin.

I feel like I have sucked all the fun out of your life. Sorry about that. Keep in mind, what works for some won't work for others. Do what's best for you and your family.

Prayers, Mantras, and Superstitions

After doing everything perfectly, timing intercourse, taking care of your body, taking vitamins and supplements, even fertility treatments, after all of that when we're still not pregnant it becomes very tempting to look to religion or the occult. I'll admit to having bought special candles, herbs, and stones, throwing coins into fountains, meditating, making wishes...everything.

If you have a religion, that's great and can be a wonderful source of comfort to you. A religious community can also be very supportive. Talk to your spiritual leader; they might have some insight or recommendations. Prayer is an important way of not just communicating with the divine, but getting in touch with yourself.

Meditation is amazing for you. It helps, especially when you're super stressed and anxious about conceiving. If you're not already practicing, then you should give it a try for five to ten minutes to start off. There are guided meditations on the internet, in your local library, and there are a ton of apps out there.

A mantra is a phrase that you repeat to yourself multiple times with intention. Some say that a mantra sends energy out into the universe, and this in turn will create the effect you desire. Others will insist that the point is to focus your attention inward. For some it is a part of their religion, for others it is a way of affirming something for themselves. Whatever the case, I feel like it works. You can choose from ancient and time-honored mantras, like *om mani padme hum* (a Sanskrit phrase that is very powerful in Buddhism), or create your own, something like *I am the mama of a happy, healthy baby* or *I can get pregnant, I will get pregnant*. Repeat, with focus, your mantra as many times as you feel like. In some traditions 108 is considered ideal, but if, for example, after you've had baby making sex you think or say your mantra five times, then five times is better than no times.

There are also hundreds of superstitions out there, with talismans to rub or days of the year to do it.

Some of my favorite:
-Don't clean under your bed (it sweeps away your baby's spirit)
-Keep a hammer under your bed for a boy
-Wear rose quartz
-Stuff a fertility stone in your bra or in your pocket
-Go on a vacation
-If you adopt, then you'll conceive
-Be cheerful; when babies choose parents they want someone who looks fun
-Put fruit seeds in a clean eggshell and bury it in your backyard
-Avoid funerals and cemeteries
-Eat pineapples right after ovulation (some science here; bromelain in the core may help)
-Receive as a gift parsley plant/seeds (but don't eat in excess)
-Drink from a pregnant woman's glass/rub her belly (if she'll let you!)
-Order your baby from the universe (via the internet); it's called cosmic ordering
-Eat a lot of fruit to bear fruit
-Eating too much parsley or sage (and some other herbs) can lead to miscarriage (some science backs this up)
-In summer, go outside and garden naked
-You'll *know* the moment you're pregnant
-A sign will appear before you get pregnant
-Avoid eclipses, both lunar and solar
-Just relax! (ok, some science, but if I hear it one more time…!)

There's an A.R.T. to It

Assisted Reproductive Technologies. Pretty much what it sounds like: using science/technology to help people conceive.

First of all, it's a good idea to come up with a timeline for yourself, to determine at what point, if any, you want to seek help. The rule of thumb is to try unprotected sex for six months if you're over 35, one year if you're under, before seeking fertility help. Technically peak fertility is in a woman's early to mid-twenties, and even then in a given month you only have about a twenty percent chance of conceiving-and that's if you and your partner/spouse are in perfect health and timing everything right!

Whether you've passed that mark or not, it's a good idea to have a plan in place. It can be tempting to rush into expensive and invasive procedures just because you're so ready to have a baby, but maybe you need to give it more time. On the flip side, you or your partner may be thinking it'll just happen, and then suddenly you realize you've been trying for over a year and something may be wrong. Talk it over with your partner/spouse, talk it over with your doctor, and come up with a plan that works for you. If you never seek out reproductive help you still may have a chance of conceiving naturally, so do what feels right for you and your family.

Ob/gyn check up: If you haven't already seen your ob/gyn about a pre-pregnancy check up, you should do so as soon as possible. They can give you valuable information about preparing your body for pregnancy and they'll give you the green light healthwise.

My plan: _____

Outcome: _____

Next step: _____

Non-invasive Fertility Tests: Semen analysis (if you have a male partner/spouse), blood work, hormone check, ultrasound, and physical exam. You might also talk to your doctor about your cycle specifically and confirm that you're tracking ovulation accurately. My doctor even examined me around ovulation to determine my cervical mucus quality and opening, which was no more invasive than a pap.

My plan: _____

Outcome: _____

Next step: _____

Fertility Drugs: Clomid/clomiphene, Letrozole/Femara, injectable hormones, progesterone supplements, estrogen supplements, metformin, birth control (to regulate cycle), herbs, vitamins, or medicine to balance another medical issue, such as increased levels of synthroid for thyroid issues.

My plan: _____

Outcome: _____

Next step: _____

Lifestyle changes: Weight gain/loss, diet/nutrition, change activity level, cut out smoking/drinking/caffeine, etc. See page 27.

My plan: _____

Outcome: _____

Next step: _____

Invasive Exams: Hysterosonogram (sonogram of uterus), hyterosalpingogram (checks for blockage in the fallopian tubes; bonus: it can lead to increased fertility for a few months), post-coital test (what it sounds like), cervical mucus test, biopsies, water ultrasound, and more.

My plan: _____

Outcome: _____

Next step: _____

Intrauterine Insemination (IUI): Your partner/spouse's semen or donor semen is specially prepped and inserted directly into your uterus, bypassing the cervix if there are issues there, getting sperm closer to your egg, and helps out with male infertility or ovulation issues. Also involves supplementary hormone injections in most cases to ensure perfect timing of procedure.

My plan: _____

Outcome: _____

Next step: _____

Invitro Fertilization (IVF): The most famous, perhaps, of fertility treatments. It boasts the highest success rates, but is also the most invasive and expensive. Essentially, your partner/spouse's or donor's sperm is joined with your egg in a lab and then medically implanted in your uterus. In some cases of unexplained fertility it can also diagnose underlying issues. Further, if you have multiple fertilized eggs implanted, which is generally recommended in women over forty, then you run the risk of multiples.

My plan: _____

Outcome: _____

Next step: _____

Corrective Surgery: For severe endometriosis, tube blockage, and other fertility issues.

My plan: _____

Outcome: _____

Next step: _____

Acupuncture and Other Alternative Treatments: Controversial, but some studies show a positive correlation between acupuncture and fertility. Be sure to seek out a licensed practioner; your doctor may have referrals for you.

My plan: _____

Outcome: _____

Next step: _____

Other Treatments: Your doctor may suggest further treatments.

My plan: _____

Outcome: _____

Next step: _____

Surrogacy: Your egg, your partner/spouse's sperm, a donor egg, donor sperm, or some combination are joined and then implanted in another woman's uterus. Another woman carries and births your baby.

My plan: _____

Outcome: _____

Next step: _____

Adoption: Some may begin the adoption process while baby is still a bun in the oven, while others may foster or adopt from any age up to eighteen. Private adoptions and adoptions through government entities are options and law varies from state to state. It is generally advisable to seek legal counsel to guide you through the adoption process.

My plan: _____

Outcome: _____

Next step: _____

Please keep in mind that these are common and typical steps to treat infertility, but it is by no means a complete list of all available options, nor will all options be right for you. You don't have to try them in this order, or do everything I've listed. I haven't used many fertility drugs, and there have been lifestyle changes that I haven't fully committed to. Again, I urge you to talk over your options with your doctor and conduct your own research before making decisions for your body and your family.

Finally, and this option may not be for you, but for some there may be a point when you stop trying. For some, it'll be after a set amount of time, for others it may be after a set number of tries with IUI or IVF. This doesn't mean you're not still coping and hoping you'll have a baby, but you might stop seeking fertility treatment. For me, I'll never not be able to note changes in cervical mucus; I'll never not hope that a slight fever a week after ovulating means I'm pregnant. But there have been times in this journey when my husband and I have decided to take a break, skip the doctor, try to conceive naturally, and focus on other things.

My plan: _____

Outcome: _____

Next step: _____

I Dream of Baby: Toddler Years

Now again, picture that little one in your mind as a toddler. I know, I know…if you're like me this might make you tear up or straight up bawl. I'm sorry, but it really helps me, it gives me hope to picture my baby as a toddler. As always, feel free to skip.

Hair color: _____

Hair texture: _____

Eye color: _____

Skin color: _____

Smile: _____

Height: _____

Weight: _____

What games will you play with your baby? _____

_____

_____

What will holidays be like? _____

_____

_____

Describe a typical day in your life, from morning until bedtime.

_____

_____

_____

_____

_____

_____

How will you start to teach your little one about the world? How will you guide them, encourage them, reprimand them? _____

_____

_____

_____

_____

Anything else you want to include:

_____

_____

If it's too hard to do, skip this part, that's fine. But remember, we're putting ourselves through all this for our little ones and sometimes visualization can lead to success.

Imagine now your child.

Describe your kiddo's first day of school. _____

_____

_____

_____

_____

How will your typical day go? _____

_____

_____

_____

_____

Will they have chores? Which ones, if so? _____

_____

_____

How will you encourage them in school? _____

_____

_____

How will you have serious conversations with them, like "the birds and the bees," dealing with loss, fitting in with peers without caving to peer pressure?

_____

_____

_____

_____

_____

What are some activities you might encourage kiddo to take part in?

_____

_____

What are some special things you'll do together, just you two?

_____

_____

_____

_____

We'll take a break from this for now, but we'll come back to the teen years and beyond. I have faith in this future.

Stories of Hope

Infertility and subfertility are much more common than we are led to believe, mostly because most of us going through it don't like to talk about it. But there are so many stories out there of people who tried for years and then went on to have whole passels of kids. Maybe you're not in the mood to hear it today, and that's just fine. But if ever you want a little more hope, here are some personal stories:

"Towards the end of 2013, my husband and I decided we wanted to start trying. So, I did what everyone suggests and got off birth control and started taking prenatal vitamins. As I was tracking, I noticed that I only ovulated 2 times in 6 months. So, I went to my primary ob. She immediately referred me to a fertility doctor instead of waiting a year since there was clearly a problem. After every test, the result was "mild" pcos. So, I started letrozole, metformin, and a trigger shot. After months of no pregnancies, we switched to IUIs. I got pregnant the first time! At the first ultrasound, our doctor told us the baby was small based on date of conception, but otherwise healthy. We got the same report at every appointment, until 12.5 weeks when our sweet girl no longer had a heart beat. That was in April. We waited a few months and tried again. We started with a couple more IUIs again with no luck. We also added additional shots to boost my lining. On the fifth IUI, I was cautiously optimistic again- but then my doctor called and said that the blood showed it was most likely not viable since the hcg was so so low. Two days later I did another blood test which showed even lower numbers; I had a chemical pregnancy [an early miscarriage]. After another month of no success, I went in for more tests and my doctor told me that she would only recommend one more IUI and then it was time to move to IVF. She also said we had to take December off from treatments because she was afraid my ovulation may coincide with Christmas. Well, we had the ultimate Christmas miracle and conceived naturally! We have a beautiful two year old daughter and every shot, tear, and heartache was worth the wait that ultimately brought her to our family."

"Our journey trying to get pregnant started a couple years after we got married. In 2012 we finally conceived naturally, but I ended up having a miscarriage when I was about 8 weeks. After that, I knew I wasn't ready to try again for a while due to all the physical and emotional pain we went through. In January 2017 we decided to go to a fertility clinic and try again. I took Clomid for 5 days and got pregnant right away. A week later after finding out about my pregnancy I had a chemical pregnancy [an early miscarriage]. I took one month off so my body could go back to normal and I got pregnant the next month with our rainbow baby Mason, who was born in April 2018."

Do you have any friends or family in a similar situation? Have you read about anyone in a book, a blog, a movie? How about a blog? Do you follow anyone on social media with a success story? Write down some stories that inspire you.

_____

_____

_____

_____

_____

Enjoying the Things Now That You Can't Do Once You Have a Baby

I'll admit it: there have been times I see a colicky baby, a screaming toddler, an out-of-control child, or rebellious teens and think, *whew! At least I don't have to deal with that*. Of course I'm completely looking forward to being a parent and I know a little bit of what that entails and it won't be all smiles and cuddles. But there are moments of, not relief, but appreciation for the life I have now, which is infinitely more manageable and convenient than it will be when I have a baby. So let's take a moment and look on the bright side.

Things you can't do once you get pregnant:
- Sleep well
- Smoke
- Drink caffeine
- Eat sushi, lunch meat, etc.
- Laying on your back
- Roller coasters
- Some travel
- Drink beer/wine/liquor
- Take medicine when you're sick
- Certain exercises
- Hot tubs/hot baths
- Eat junk food (well, maybe)

Plus, you'll be sore, tired, nauseous, moody, and you'll have to pee all the time.

Things can't do once you have a little kid (at least not easily):
- Do what you want when you want to do it
- Watch what tv you want to watch
- Swear
- Travel
- Go out all night
- Listen to the music you want
- Sleep

And you'll have to change diapers, do more laundry, clean, cook more, and, you know, be responsible for a life.

The Worst Advice

The one we all hear the most is: "just relax!" Ugh. As a friend once said of this: "would you tell someone with any other medical issue to 'just relax'? No!" People with diabetes are told to seek treatment, not to relax; cancer patients are given medicine, not a prescription to calm down; even if you catch a cold you're told to intake fluids, take cold medicine, get extra sleep, take zinc or vitamin c. No, infertility/subfertility is not the same as cancer. But it's hella insensitive for people, especially those with children, to treat us like we're being hysterical, like it's all in our heads.

"When you're really ready, it'll happen." *Excuse me?*

"Try *fill-in-the-blank-medical-treatment*." Are you a doctor? Are you my doctor? No! Maybe the drug you're recommending would be bad for me. Maybe I can't afford the procedure you're suggesting.

"Oh you should stop eating this and drinking that," where this and that are foods and drinks you really want. I know I'm being a hypocrite here, because I kind of am doing that to you a little, but you know what I mean, right?

"Stop trying and it'll just happen." It is impossible, once you're on baby journey, to stop trying. Maybe I can throw away my charts or quit fertility treatments, but I will always want a baby, because once I decided to have a baby, in my mind I became a mother and until my baby comes home to me my life will be missing something.

"Trust your intuition." Uh, maybe your intuition should have told you not to say something so insensitive. It's. Not. My. Fault.

How to Deal With Awkward Questions

Because it's going to happen. Some nosy person, who has no business asking you such personal questions, will do so. Ugh.

The most common: "You're of-a-certain-age/you've been married a-certain-amount-of-time: when are you going to have a baby?" A. None of your business. B. None of your business. But how to respond? If it's someone you know and are comfortable with, you can say the generous and patient response: "we've been trying, coping, and hoping for x amount of time." The problem with that is, it tends to lead to advice or sympathy. The few times I've told that truth to people I get, "oh it'll happen," if I'm lucky, otherwise I get versions of everything I listed on page 46. Ugh, again.

> Some other possible responses to try:
> -I can't have children, but thank you for asking (makes the asker super uncomfortable and they change the subject)
> -Oh, thank you! Could you please explain how it all works?
> -It's in God's hands now
> -Confuse them, i.e. I once quoted *A Game of Thrones* and said "When the sun rises in the west and sets in the east..."

It can be kind of fun to see what elicits different responses, but in all seriousness: I do not tell people I'm trying to conceive, because it leads to conversations I don't want to have. But, sometimes it's unavoidable. I've used all of the above, but generally I say "one of these days," or "maybe," then I change the subject.

"Have you tried such and such?" Everyone thinks they know the answer, that they will be the one to solve your infertility.

> -Thank you, I'll mention it to my doctor-it's polite and final
> -I'll keep that in mind, thank you
> -We're going to do this our way, but thank you

-Have you tried minding your own business?-okay, this
one's not so polite

-Interesting, thanks, we'll have to give that a try

If you can, try to keep in mind: they really do think they're trying
to help you. They just don't understand. Try to explain it to them,
or ask them to do a little research about how to talk to you about
this. You could send them a copy of Meg Keys's *The Waiting Line-
What to Do (and Not Do) When Someone You Love is Dealing with
Infertility* as a good resource for how to best support you. Or as a
not-so-subtle-hint that what they're saying is hurtful.

What have you heard and how did you respond?

Awkward Question 1: _____

_____

Response: _____

A.Q. 2: _____

Response: _____

_____

A.Q. 3: _____

Response: _____

_____

Teen Years

If you don't like doing this part of the journal, feel free to skip, of course. But now we'll picture baby in their teen years.

Describe your teen physically (again, it can be useful to picture yourself or your partner/spouse as a teen): _____

_____

_____

_____

_____

What activities are they into? _____

_____

_____

What is school like for them, what are their grades like? Are they preparing to go to college or into a trade?

_____

_____

_____

_____

What are some things the two of you do together? _____

_____

_____

_____

How do you deal with any teenage rebellion? _____

_____

_____

_____

Describe some milestone events or rights of passage, such as driving a car, graduation, prom, first dates, etc.

_____

_____

_____

_____

_____

_____

_____

Grown Up Kids

Here's hoping that someday, years down the road, this journey, this trial, this journal, will be behind you and you'll have watched your little baby grown into the amazing person they'll be. This is the final entry for imagining your baby at different times in their lives. It's tough, but again: the point of this exercise is to remember why all the pain and waiting is worth it.

Describe your grown up: _____

_____

_____

Are they married? Do they have kids? A house? What does their life look like? _____

_____

_____

_____

_____

Picture them in a generic profession (I mean, don't choose a job for them already, but imagine some of the shared aspects of all jobs, like being at a computer, talking to people, commuting).

_____

_____

What are some things you do together? _____

_____

_____

_____

What are holidays like now? _____

_____

_____

_____

Anything else you want to add: _____

_____

_____

_____

_____

_____

_____

_____

Name That Baby!

It's fun and I can't help it. I already have a list of baby names.
Keep your list here so you can add some and maybe occasionally
cross one out. If you feel like one name is more middle-name
material then put it in parenthesis. If there's one you especially
like, mark it by putting a little star next to it.

Girl Names   Boy Names

_____   _____

_____   _____

_____   _____

_____   _____

_____   _____

_____   _____

_____   _____

_____   _____

Names that could be used for either/both:

_____

_____

Letter To Baby

I've seen in pregnancy books a place for mothers-to-be to write to their unborn child, all the love and wisdom that is in their hearts, all their thoughts about pregnancy and their expectations for the future. Well, why not us? Write to your baby and tell him/her/them all the wonderful ways you'll love them, the life they have to look forward to, and what you're going through now.

Date: _____

Dear _____,

_____

_____

_____

_____

_____

_____

_____

_____

_____

The Doctors: Fertility, ObGyn, and GP

One of the most frustrating parts of infertility is feeling like you don't have any control. Doctors sometimes exacerbate that feeling for me. My doctors have done test after test, but never go over the results, except a quick phone call saying "it's good enough," or, even when they do follow up, they never explain what the first one said. Literally during my HSG (Hysterosalpingogram -it checks for blocks in your fallopian tubes- it's very uncomfortable and pretty darn invasive) the nurse said "oh and we got your husband's semen analysis. It's fine, just tell him to take a multivitamin." Really? That's all the feedback? My feet were in stirrups and I was naked from the waist down and this is when they tell me?

Do your research! Know what they're doing to your body when they say they're running a test. Then ask for the results, preferably in person. What I ended up doing was having my fertility specialist send the results to my regular ob/gyn, had them upload the results to an online account, and then went over the data, using the internet to interpret and translate. Then I had my ob/gyn go over the results with me. It seems like a lot of steps, and it is, but it's worth it to me. Hopefully you have doctors that are good at communicating.

Whatever the case may be, it's important for you to do your homework, to advocate for yourself. Keep notes in your journal, plus questions you may have, alternatives you may want to try, and then take notes at your doctor's office. If they're rushing you, you may need to find another doctor. This is important. This is your baby. This is your life.

This goes for regular check-ups. The body does not work in isolation, so it's good to have an annual wellness exam, and all of the stuff they're testing may be impacting your fertility, including blood pressure (high and low), thyroid, inflammation, vitamin deficiency...if your body isn't healthy, it's not going to divest resources to making a baby.

Questions:

Date	Question	Doctor's Answer

Date	Question	Doctor's Answer

Date	Question	Doctor's Answer

Date	Question	Doctor's Answer

Notes from Doctor's Appointment:

Date	Doctor	Notes

Notes from Doctor's Appointment:

Date	Doctor	Notes

Notes from Doctor's Appointment:

Date	Doctor	Notes

Notes from Doctor's Appointment:

Date	Doctor	Notes

Notes from Doctor's Appointment:

Date	Doctor	Notes

Journal break-down-

Day of cycle: Day one is your first day of flow (not spotting). Count onward through your cycle until the next day of flow, and then start over. Or, if you're pregnant shelve this book for when you have a passel of kids around you and then you can throw it away, read it for nostalgia, whatever.

What's going on in my cycle: This is what part of your cycle you're in. Options: spotting, period, spotting, follicular (you're not on your period, but you haven't ovulated yet), fertile (as determine by cervical mucus, pee kits, fertility monitors, cervical opening, etc.), ovulating, and luteal (between when you ovulated and when your next period comes).

Symptoms: Describe what your physical body is feeling or any unusual occurrences (for example, I dream a lot more in my luteal phase. Weird, but true).

Exercise and nutrition: Most sources suggest mild physical activity, such as walking, swimming, and yoga. Rigorous sports and exercises are thought to negatively impact fertility. What you eat can also affect your fertility to some degree. There's an awful lot of debate out there about organic food, the effects of dairy, meat consumption, carbs, sugar, added sugar, processed foods. See pages 27-29 for more information. All that's really locked down is that being a healthy weight increases your odds. That means different things for everybody! If you suddenly gain or lose a bunch of weight that's going to throw your system off, so take it easy. Record what you're eating in this box and look for a pattern. If you've tried one diet for a few months and you're not pregnant, maybe try something new gradually. That being said, I've tried just about ever recommended vitamin supplement (COQ10, Bromelain, wheatgrass, D, E...the list is endless). All they did was make me feel nauseous, which got my hopes up that I was pregnant, but I wasn't, I was just sick. The only supplement I really put my faith in is cinnamon. One teeny tiny but strong study showed that it helps with ovulation. When I'm eating cinnamon I notice that my cycle is more regular. It could be a placebo effect, but even if it is, hey, that still means it's working.

My thoughts/feelings: Pretty self-explanatory and self-guided. Vent, hope, make a wish, make notes about something you read online...anything you want. It can be for your eyes only, or a way for you to communicate what you're going through to a spouse/partner, your family, and your friends. I've never kept a journal before, so I found it helped me to address it to my baby.

Prenatal vitamin check: From the moment you start trying to conceive (or earlier!) you should be taking a prenatal vitamin (talk to your doctor; as stated, I'm not a medical professional and this advice should be treated as such). Try to take it at the same time every day, but if there are conflicts or if you're prone to forgetting then give it a check mark every day. There's also a spot for other medicines, depending on what you have to take, especially if you are prescribed fertility medication by your doctor.

The chart space is for recording your daily basal body temperature, cervical mucus, cervical opening, and additional notes.

A final note before I turn the rest of the writing in this book over to you. I know how awful this is and I am so sorry that you're suffering, too. I hope in some way this book has helped you, because writing it really has been such a comfort to me. Warm wishes, best of luck, and lots of love.

Day of Cycle:	Date:

What's going on in my cycle:

Symptoms:

Exercise and Nutrition:

BBT:	CM:	CO:

Notes:

My thoughts/feelings:

_____

_____

_____

_____

_____

_____

_____

_____

_____

_____

_____

Prenatal Vitamin Check:	Other medicine:

Day of Cycle: Date:
What's going on in my cycle:
Symptoms:
Exercise and Nutrition:
BBT: CM: CO: Notes:
My thoughts/feelings:

_____

_____

_____

_____

_____

_____

_____

_____

_____

_____

_____

_____

Prenatal Vitamin Check: Other medicine:

Day of Cycle: Date:

What's going on in my cycle:

Symptoms:

Exercise and Nutrition:

BBT: CM: CO:

Notes:

My thoughts/feelings:

_____

_____

_____

_____

_____

_____

_____

_____

_____

_____

Prenatal Vitamin Check: Other medicine:

Day of Cycle:	Date:

What's going on in my cycle:

Symptoms:

Exercise and Nutrition:

BBT: CM: CO:

Notes:

My thoughts/feelings:

_____

_____

_____

_____

_____

_____

_____

_____

_____

_____

_____

Prenatal Vitamin Check: Other medicine:

Day of Cycle:	Date:

What's going on in my cycle:

Symptoms:

Exercise and Nutrition:

BBT: CM: CO:
Notes:

My thoughts/feelings:

_____

_____

_____

_____

_____

_____

_____

_____

_____

_____

_____

Prenatal Vitamin Check: Other medicine:

Day of Cycle: Date:

What's going on in my cycle:

Symptoms:

Exercise and Nutrition:

BBT: CM: CO:
Notes:

My thoughts/feelings:

_____

_____

_____

_____

_____

_____

_____

_____

_____

_____

_____

Prenatal Vitamin Check: Other medicine:

Day of Cycle: Date:

What's going on in my cycle:

Symptoms:

Exercise and Nutrition:

BBT: CM: CO:

Notes:

My thoughts/feelings:

_____

_____

_____

_____

_____

_____

_____

_____

_____

_____

Prenatal Vitamin Check: Other medicine:

Day of Cycle: Date:

What's going on in my cycle:

Symptoms:

Exercise and Nutrition:

BBT: CM: CO:
Notes:

My thoughts/feelings:

_____

_____

_____

_____

_____

_____

_____

_____

_____

_____

_____

Prenatal Vitamin Check: Other medicine:

Day of Cycle:	Date:

What's going on in my cycle:

Symptoms:

Exercise and Nutrition:

BBT: CM: CO:

Notes:

My thoughts/feelings:

_____

_____

_____

_____

_____

_____

_____

_____

_____

_____

_____

Prenatal Vitamin Check: Other medicine:

Day of Cycle: Date:

What's going on in my cycle:

Symptoms:

Exercise and Nutrition:

BBT: CM: CO:
Notes:

My thoughts/feelings:

_____

_____

_____

_____

_____

_____

_____

_____

_____

_____

_____

Prenatal Vitamin Check: Other medicine:

Day of Cycle:	Date:

What's going on in my cycle:

Symptoms:

Exercise and Nutrition:

BBT: CM: CO:

Notes:

My thoughts/feelings:

_____

_____

_____

_____

_____

_____

_____

_____

_____

_____

Prenatal Vitamin Check: Other medicine:

Day of Cycle: Date:

What's going on in my cycle:

Symptoms:

Exercise and Nutrition:

BBT: CM: CO:
Notes:

My thoughts/feelings:

_____

_____

_____

_____

_____

_____

_____

_____

_____

_____

_____

Prenatal Vitamin Check: Other medicine:

Day of Cycle:	Date:

What's going on in my cycle:

Symptoms:

Exercise and Nutrition:

BBT: CM: CO:
Notes:

My thoughts/feelings:

_____

_____

_____

_____

_____

_____

_____

_____

_____

_____

_____

Prenatal Vitamin Check: Other medicine:

Day of Cycle:	Date:

What's going on in my cycle:

Symptoms:

Exercise and Nutrition:

BBT: CM: CO:
Notes:

My thoughts/feelings:

_____

_____

_____

_____

_____

_____

_____

_____

_____

_____

_____

Prenatal Vitamin Check: Other medicine:

Day of Cycle: Date:

What's going on in my cycle:

Symptoms:

Exercise and Nutrition:

BBT: CM: CO:
Notes:

My thoughts/feelings:

_____

_____

_____

_____

_____

_____

_____

_____

_____

_____

Prenatal Vitamin Check: Other medicine:

Day of Cycle:	Date:

What's going on in my cycle:

Symptoms:

Exercise and Nutrition:

BBT: CM: CO:
Notes:

My thoughts/feelings:

_____

_____

_____

_____

_____

_____

_____

_____

_____

_____

_____

Prenatal Vitamin Check: Other medicine:

Day of Cycle: Date:

What's going on in my cycle:

Symptoms:

Exercise and Nutrition:

BBT: CM: CO:
Notes:

My thoughts/feelings:

_____

_____

_____

_____

_____

_____

_____

_____

_____

_____

Prenatal Vitamin Check: Other medicine:

Day of Cycle: Date:

What's going on in my cycle:

Symptoms:

Exercise and Nutrition:

BBT: CM: CO:
Notes:

My thoughts/feelings:

_____

_____

_____

_____

_____

_____

_____

_____

_____

_____

Prenatal Vitamin Check: Other medicine:

Day of Cycle:	Date:

What's going on in my cycle:

Symptoms:

Exercise and Nutrition:

BBT: CM: CO:

Notes:

My thoughts/feelings:

_____

_____

_____

_____

_____

_____

_____

_____

_____

_____

Prenatal Vitamin Check: Other medicine:

Day of Cycle:	Date:

What's going on in my cycle:

Symptoms:

Exercise and Nutrition:

BBT: CM: CO:
Notes:

My thoughts/feelings:

_____

_____

_____

_____

_____

_____

_____

_____

_____

_____

Prenatal Vitamin Check: Other medicine:

Day of Cycle:	Date:

What's going on in my cycle:

Symptoms:

Exercise and Nutrition:

BBT: CM: CO:
Notes:

My thoughts/feelings:

_____

_____

_____

_____

_____

_____

_____

_____

_____

_____

Prenatal Vitamin Check: Other medicine:

Day of Cycle: Date:

What's going on in my cycle:

Symptoms:

Exercise and Nutrition:

BBT: CM: CO:
Notes:

My thoughts/feelings:

_____

_____

_____

_____

_____

_____

_____

_____

_____

_____

_____

Prenatal Vitamin Check: Other medicine:

Day of Cycle: Date:

What's going on in my cycle:

Symptoms:

Exercise and Nutrition:

BBT: CM: CO:

Notes:

My thoughts/feelings:

_____

_____

_____

_____

_____

_____

_____

_____

_____

_____

_____

Prenatal Vitamin Check: Other medicine:

Day of Cycle: Date:

What's going on in my cycle:

Symptoms:

Exercise and Nutrition:

BBT: CM: CO:
Notes:

My thoughts/feelings:

_____

_____

_____

_____

_____

_____

_____

_____

_____

_____

_____

Prenatal Vitamin Check: Other medicine:

Day of Cycle:	Date:

What's going on in my cycle:

Symptoms:

Exercise and Nutrition:

BBT:　　　　　　CM:　　　　　　CO:
Notes:

My thoughts/feelings:

_____

_____

_____

_____

_____

_____

_____

_____

_____

_____

Prenatal Vitamin Check:　　　　Other medicine:

Day of Cycle: Date:

What's going on in my cycle:

Symptoms:

Exercise and Nutrition:

BBT: CM: CO:
Notes:

My thoughts/feelings:

_____

_____

_____

_____

_____

_____

_____

_____

_____

_____

_____

Prenatal Vitamin Check: Other medicine:

Day of Cycle: Date:

What's going on in my cycle:

Symptoms:

Exercise and Nutrition:

BBT: CM: CO:

Notes:

My thoughts/feelings:

_____

_____

_____

_____

_____

_____

_____

_____

_____

_____

_____

Prenatal Vitamin Check: Other medicine:

Day of Cycle: Date:

What's going on in my cycle:

Symptoms:

Exercise and Nutrition:

BBT: CM: CO:
Notes:

My thoughts/feelings:

_____

_____

_____

_____

_____

_____

_____

_____

_____

_____

_____

Prenatal Vitamin Check: Other medicine:

Day of Cycle: Date:

What's going on in my cycle:

Symptoms:

Exercise and Nutrition:

BBT: CM: CO:
Notes:

My thoughts/feelings:

_____

_____

_____

_____

_____

_____

_____

_____

_____

_____

_____

Prenatal Vitamin Check: Other medicine:

Day of Cycle: Date:

What's going on in my cycle:

Symptoms:

Exercise and Nutrition:

BBT: CM: CO:
Notes:

My thoughts/feelings:

_____

_____

_____

_____

_____

_____

_____

_____

_____

_____

_____

Prenatal Vitamin Check: Other medicine:

Day of Cycle:	Date:

What's going on in my cycle:

Symptoms:

Exercise and Nutrition:

BBT: CM: CO:
Notes:

My thoughts/feelings:

_____

_____

_____

_____

_____

_____

_____

_____

_____

_____

Prenatal Vitamin Check:	Other medicine:

Day of Cycle: Date:

What's going on in my cycle:

Symptoms:

Exercise and Nutrition:

BBT: CM: CO:
Notes:

My thoughts/feelings:

_____

_____

_____

_____

_____

_____

_____

_____

_____

_____

Prenatal Vitamin Check: Other medicine:

Day of Cycle:	Date:

What's going on in my cycle:

Symptoms:

Exercise and Nutrition:

BBT: CM: CO:

Notes:

My thoughts/feelings:

_____

_____

_____

_____

_____

_____

_____

_____

_____

_____

_____

Prenatal Vitamin Check: Other medicine:

Day of Cycle:	Date:

What's going on in my cycle:

Symptoms:

Exercise and Nutrition:

BBT: CM: CO:
Notes:

My thoughts/feelings:

_____

_____

_____

_____

_____

_____

_____

_____

_____

_____

Prenatal Vitamin Check: Other medicine:

Day of Cycle: Date:

What's going on in my cycle:

Symptoms:

Exercise and Nutrition:

BBT: CM: CO:
Notes:

My thoughts/feelings:

_____

_____

_____

_____

_____

_____

_____

_____

_____

_____

Prenatal Vitamin Check: Other medicine:

Day of Cycle: Date:

What's going on in my cycle:

Symptoms:

Exercise and Nutrition:

BBT: CM: CO:

Notes:

My thoughts/feelings:

_____

_____

_____

_____

_____

_____

_____

_____

_____

_____

_____

Prenatal Vitamin Check: Other medicine:

Day of Cycle: Date:

What's going on in my cycle:

Symptoms:

Exercise and Nutrition:

BBT: CM: CO:

Notes:

My thoughts/feelings:

_____

_____

_____

_____

_____

_____

_____

_____

_____

_____

_____

Prenatal Vitamin Check: Other medicine:

Day of Cycle: Date:

What's going on in my cycle:

Symptoms:

Exercise and Nutrition:

BBT: CM: CO:

Notes:

My thoughts/feelings:

_____

_____

_____

_____

_____

_____

_____

_____

_____

_____

_____

Prenatal Vitamin Check: Other medicine:

Day of Cycle: Date:

What's going on in my cycle:

Symptoms:

Exercise and Nutrition:

BBT: CM: CO:
Notes:

My thoughts/feelings:

_____

_____

_____

_____

_____

_____

_____

_____

_____

_____

_____

Prenatal Vitamin Check: Other medicine:

Day of Cycle:	Date:

What's going on in my cycle:

Symptoms:

Exercise and Nutrition:

BBT: CM: CO:
Notes:

My thoughts/feelings:

_____

_____

_____

_____

_____

_____

_____

_____

_____

_____

Prenatal Vitamin Check: Other medicine:

Day of Cycle: Date:

What's going on in my cycle:

Symptoms:

Exercise and Nutrition:

BBT: CM: CO:
Notes:

My thoughts/feelings:

_____

_____

_____

_____

_____

_____

_____

_____

_____

_____

_____

Prenatal Vitamin Check: Other medicine:

Day of Cycle: Date:

What's going on in my cycle:

Symptoms:

Exercise and Nutrition:

BBT: CM: CO:
Notes:

My thoughts/feelings:

_____

_____

_____

_____

_____

_____

_____

_____

_____

_____

Prenatal Vitamin Check: Other medicine:

Day of Cycle:	Date:

What's going on in my cycle:

Symptoms:

Exercise and Nutrition:

BBT: CM: CO:
Notes:

My thoughts/feelings:

_____

_____

_____

_____

_____

_____

_____

_____

_____

_____

Prenatal Vitamin Check: Other medicine:

Day of Cycle:	Date:

What's going on in my cycle:

Symptoms:

Exercise and Nutrition:

BBT:	CM:	CO:

Notes:

My thoughts/feelings:

_____

_____

_____

_____

_____

_____

_____

_____

_____

_____

_____

Prenatal Vitamin Check:	Other medicine:

Day of Cycle:	Date:

What's going on in my cycle:

Symptoms:

Exercise and Nutrition:

BBT: CM: CO:

Notes:

My thoughts/feelings:

_____

_____

_____

_____

_____

_____

_____

_____

_____

_____

Prenatal Vitamin Check: Other medicine:

Day of Cycle:	Date:

What's going on in my cycle:

Symptoms:

Exercise and Nutrition:

BBT: CM: CO:
Notes:

My thoughts/feelings:

_____

_____

_____

_____

_____

_____

_____

_____

_____

_____

_____

Prenatal Vitamin Check: Other medicine:

Day of Cycle: Date:

What's going on in my cycle:

Symptoms:

Exercise and Nutrition:

BBT: CM: CO:
Notes:

My thoughts/feelings:

_____

_____

_____

_____

_____

_____

_____

_____

_____

_____

_____

Prenatal Vitamin Check: Other medicine:

Day of Cycle: Date:

What's going on in my cycle:

Symptoms:

Exercise and Nutrition:

BBT: CM: CO:
Notes:

My thoughts/feelings:

_____

_____

_____

_____

_____

_____

_____

_____

_____

_____

Prenatal Vitamin Check: Other medicine:

Day of Cycle:	Date:

What's going on in my cycle:

Symptoms:

Exercise and Nutrition:

BBT:	CM:	CO:

Notes:

My thoughts/feelings:

_____

_____

_____

_____

_____

_____

_____

_____

_____

_____

_____

Prenatal Vitamin Check:	Other medicine:

Day of Cycle: Date:

What's going on in my cycle:

Symptoms:

Exercise and Nutrition:

BBT: CM: CO:

Notes:

My thoughts/feelings:

_____

_____

_____

_____

_____

_____

_____

_____

_____

_____

_____

Prenatal Vitamin Check: Other medicine:

Day of Cycle: Date:

What's going on in my cycle:

Symptoms:

Exercise and Nutrition:

BBT: CM: CO:
Notes:

My thoughts/feelings:

_____

_____

_____

_____

_____

_____

_____

_____

_____

_____

_____

_____

Prenatal Vitamin Check: Other medicine:

Day of Cycle: Date:

What's going on in my cycle:

Symptoms:

Exercise and Nutrition:

BBT: CM: CO:
Notes:

My thoughts/feelings:

_____

_____

_____

_____

_____

_____

_____

_____

_____

_____

_____

Prenatal Vitamin Check: Other medicine:

Day of Cycle: Date:

What's going on in my cycle:

Symptoms:

Exercise and Nutrition:

BBT: CM: CO:
Notes:

My thoughts/feelings:

_____

_____

_____

_____

_____

_____

_____

_____

_____

_____

Prenatal Vitamin Check: Other medicine:

Day of Cycle: Date:

What's going on in my cycle:

Symptoms:

Exercise and Nutrition:

BBT: CM: CO:
Notes:

My thoughts/feelings:

_____

_____

_____

_____

_____

_____

_____

_____

_____

_____

_____

Prenatal Vitamin Check: Other medicine:

Day of Cycle:	Date:

What's going on in my cycle:

Symptoms:

Exercise and Nutrition:

BBT: CM: CO:
Notes:

My thoughts/feelings:

_____

_____

_____

_____

_____

_____

_____

_____

_____

_____

Prenatal Vitamin Check: Other medicine:

Day of Cycle: Date:

What's going on in my cycle:

Symptoms:

Exercise and Nutrition:

BBT: CM: CO:

Notes:

My thoughts/feelings:

_____

_____

_____

_____

_____

_____

_____

_____

_____

_____

_____

Prenatal Vitamin Check: Other medicine:

| Day of Cycle: | Date: |

What's going on in my cycle:

Symptoms:

Exercise and Nutrition:

BBT: CM: CO:
Notes:

My thoughts/feelings:

_____

_____

_____

_____

_____

_____

_____

_____

_____

_____

_____

Prenatal Vitamin Check: Other medicine:

Day of Cycle: Date:

What's going on in my cycle:

Symptoms:

Exercise and Nutrition:

BBT: CM: CO:

Notes:

My thoughts/feelings:

_____

_____

_____

_____

_____

_____

_____

_____

_____

_____

_____

Prenatal Vitamin Check: Other medicine:

Day of Cycle:	Date:

What's going on in my cycle:

Symptoms:

Exercise and Nutrition:

BBT: CM: CO:

Notes:

My thoughts/feelings:

_____

_____

_____

_____

_____

_____

_____

_____

_____

_____

Prenatal Vitamin Check: Other medicine:

Day of Cycle: Date:

What's going on in my cycle:

Symptoms:

Exercise and Nutrition:

BBT: CM: CO:

Notes:

My thoughts/feelings:

_____

_____

_____

_____

_____

_____

_____

_____

_____

_____

Prenatal Vitamin Check: Other medicine:

Day of Cycle: Date:

What's going on in my cycle:

Symptoms:

Exercise and Nutrition:

BBT: CM: CO:
Notes:

My thoughts/feelings:

_____

_____

_____

_____

_____

_____

_____

_____

_____

_____

Prenatal Vitamin Check: Other medicine:

Day of Cycle: Date:

What's going on in my cycle:

Symptoms:

Exercise and Nutrition:

BBT: CM: CO:
Notes:

My thoughts/feelings:

_____

_____

_____

_____

_____

_____

_____

_____

_____

_____

_____

Prenatal Vitamin Check: Other medicine:

Day of Cycle: Date:

What's going on in my cycle:

Symptoms:

Exercise and Nutrition:

BBT: CM: CO:
Notes:

My thoughts/feelings:

_____

_____

_____

_____

_____

_____

_____

_____

_____

Prenatal Vitamin Check: Other medicine:

Day of Cycle: Date:

What's going on in my cycle:

Symptoms:

Exercise and Nutrition:

BBT: CM: CO:

Notes:

My thoughts/feelings:

_____

_____

_____

_____

_____

_____

_____

_____

_____

_____

_____

Prenatal Vitamin Check: Other medicine:

Day of Cycle:	Date:

What's going on in my cycle:

Symptoms:

Exercise and Nutrition:

BBT:　　　　　　CM:　　　　　　CO:

Notes:

My thoughts/feelings:

_____

_____

_____

_____

_____

_____

_____

_____

_____

_____

_____

Prenatal Vitamin Check:　　　　　Other medicine:

Day of Cycle: Date:

What's going on in my cycle:

Symptoms:

Exercise and Nutrition:

BBT: CM: CO:
Notes:

My thoughts/feelings:

_____

_____

_____

_____

_____

_____

_____

_____

_____

_____

Prenatal Vitamin Check: Other medicine:

Day of Cycle: Date:

What's going on in my cycle:

Symptoms:

Exercise and Nutrition:

BBT: CM: CO:
Notes:

My thoughts/feelings:

_____

_____

_____

_____

_____

_____

_____

_____

_____

_____

Prenatal Vitamin Check: Other medicine:

Day of Cycle:	Date:

What's going on in my cycle:

Symptoms:

Exercise and Nutrition:

BBT: CM: CO:
Notes:

My thoughts/feelings:

_____

_____

_____

_____

_____

_____

_____

_____

_____

_____

Prenatal Vitamin Check: Other medicine:

Day of Cycle: Date:

What's going on in my cycle:

Symptoms:

Exercise and Nutrition:

BBT: CM: CO:
Notes:

My thoughts/feelings:

_____

_____

_____

_____

_____

_____

_____

_____

_____

_____

_____

Prenatal Vitamin Check: Other medicine:

Day of Cycle:	Date:

What's going on in my cycle:

Symptoms:

Exercise and Nutrition:

BBT: CM: CO:
Notes:

My thoughts/feelings:

_____

_____

_____

_____

_____

_____

_____

_____

_____

_____

Prenatal Vitamin Check: Other medicine:

Day of Cycle: Date:

What's going on in my cycle:

Symptoms:

Exercise and Nutrition:

BBT: CM: CO:
Notes:

My thoughts/feelings:

_____

_____

_____

_____

_____

_____

_____

_____

_____

_____

Prenatal Vitamin Check: Other medicine:

Day of Cycle: Date:

What's going on in my cycle:

Symptoms:

Exercise and Nutrition:

BBT: CM: CO:
Notes:

My thoughts/feelings:

_____

_____

_____

_____

_____

_____

_____

_____

_____

_____

_____

Prenatal Vitamin Check: Other medicine:

Day of Cycle:	Date:

What's going on in my cycle:

Symptoms:

Exercise and Nutrition:

BBT: CM: CO:

Notes:

My thoughts/feelings:

_____

_____

_____

_____

_____

_____

_____

_____

_____

_____

_____

Prenatal Vitamin Check: Other medicine:

Day of Cycle:	Date:

What's going on in my cycle:

Symptoms:

Exercise and Nutrition:

BBT: CM: CO:

Notes:

My thoughts/feelings:

_____

_____

_____

_____

_____

_____

_____

_____

_____

_____

_____

Prenatal Vitamin Check: Other medicine:

Day of Cycle: Date:

What's going on in my cycle:

Symptoms:

Exercise and Nutrition:

BBT: CM: CO:

Notes:

My thoughts/feelings:

_____

_____

_____

_____

_____

_____

_____

_____

_____

_____

_____

Prenatal Vitamin Check: Other medicine:

Day of Cycle:	Date:

What's going on in my cycle:

Symptoms:

Exercise and Nutrition:

BBT:　　　　　　CM:　　　　　　CO:
Notes:

My thoughts/feelings:

_____

_____

_____

_____

_____

_____

_____

_____

_____

_____

Prenatal Vitamin Check:　　　　　Other medicine:

Day of Cycle: Date:

What's going on in my cycle:

Symptoms:

Exercise and Nutrition:

BBT: CM: CO:
Notes:

My thoughts/feelings:

_____

_____

_____

_____

_____

_____

_____

_____

_____

_____

_____

Prenatal Vitamin Check: Other medicine:

Day of Cycle: Date:

What's going on in my cycle:

Symptoms:

Exercise and Nutrition:

BBT: CM: CO:
Notes:

My thoughts/feelings:

_____

_____

_____

_____

_____

_____

_____

_____

_____

_____

Prenatal Vitamin Check: Other medicine:

Day of Cycle:	Date:

What's going on in my cycle:

Symptoms:

Exercise and Nutrition:

BBT: CM: CO:

Notes:

My thoughts/feelings:

_____

_____

_____

_____

_____

_____

_____

_____

_____

_____

Prenatal Vitamin Check: Other medicine:

Day of Cycle:	Date:

What's going on in my cycle:

Symptoms:

Exercise and Nutrition:

BBT: CM: CO:

Notes:

My thoughts/feelings:

_____

_____

_____

_____

_____

_____

_____

_____

_____

_____

Prenatal Vitamin Check: Other medicine:

Day of Cycle: Date:

What's going on in my cycle:

Symptoms:

Exercise and Nutrition:

BBT: CM: CO:
Notes:

My thoughts/feelings:

_____

_____

_____

_____

_____

_____

_____

_____

_____

_____

Prenatal Vitamin Check: Other medicine:

Day of Cycle:	Date:

What's going on in my cycle:

Symptoms:

Exercise and Nutrition:

BBT: CM: CO:

Notes:

My thoughts/feelings:

_____

_____

_____

_____

_____

_____

_____

_____

_____

Prenatal Vitamin Check: Other medicine:

Day of Cycle: Date:

What's going on in my cycle:

Symptoms:

Exercise and Nutrition:

BBT: CM: CO:
Notes:

My thoughts/feelings:

_____

_____

_____

_____

_____

_____

_____

_____

_____

_____

Prenatal Vitamin Check: Other medicine:

Day of Cycle:	Date:

What's going on in my cycle:

Symptoms:

Exercise and Nutrition:

BBT:	CM:	CO:

Notes:

My thoughts/feelings:

_____

_____

_____

_____

_____

_____

_____

_____

_____

_____

Prenatal Vitamin Check:	Other medicine:

Day of Cycle:	Date:

What's going on in my cycle:

Symptoms:

Exercise and Nutrition:

BBT:　　　　　CM:　　　　　CO:

Notes:

My thoughts/feelings:

_____

_____

_____

_____

_____

_____

_____

_____

_____

_____

Prenatal Vitamin Check:　　　　　Other medicine:

Day of Cycle:	Date:

What's going on in my cycle:

Symptoms:

Exercise and Nutrition:

BBT: CM: CO:
Notes:

My thoughts/feelings:

_____

_____

_____

_____

_____

_____

_____

_____

_____

_____

Prenatal Vitamin Check: Other medicine:

Day of Cycle: Date:

What's going on in my cycle:

Symptoms:

Exercise and Nutrition:

BBT: CM: CO:
Notes:

My thoughts/feelings:

_____

_____

_____

_____

_____

_____

_____

_____

_____

_____

Prenatal Vitamin Check: Other medicine:

Day of Cycle:	Date:

What's going on in my cycle:

Symptoms:

Exercise and Nutrition:

BBT: CM: CO:
Notes:

My thoughts/feelings:

_____

_____

_____

_____

_____

_____

_____

_____

_____

_____

_____

Prenatal Vitamin Check: Other medicine:

Day of Cycle:	Date:

What's going on in my cycle:

Symptoms:

Exercise and Nutrition:

BBT: CM: CO:
Notes:

My thoughts/feelings:

_____

_____

_____

_____

_____

_____

_____

_____

_____

_____

Prenatal Vitamin Check: Other medicine:

Day of Cycle: Date:

What's going on in my cycle:

Symptoms:

Exercise and Nutrition:

BBT: CM: CO:
Notes:

My thoughts/feelings:

_____

_____

_____

_____

_____

_____

_____

_____

_____

_____

_____

Prenatal Vitamin Check: Other medicine:

Day of Cycle: Date:

What's going on in my cycle:

Symptoms:

Exercise and Nutrition:

BBT: CM: CO:
Notes:

My thoughts/feelings:

_____

_____

_____

_____

_____

_____

_____

_____

_____

_____

_____

Prenatal Vitamin Check: Other medicine:

Day of Cycle:	Date:

What's going on in my cycle:

Symptoms:

Exercise and Nutrition:

BBT: CM: CO:
Notes:

My thoughts/feelings:

_____

_____

_____

_____

_____

_____

_____

_____

_____

_____

Prenatal Vitamin Check: Other medicine:

Day of Cycle: Date:

What's going on in my cycle:

Symptoms:

Exercise and Nutrition:

BBT: CM: CO:
Notes:

My thoughts/feelings:

_____

_____

_____

_____

_____

_____

_____

_____

_____

_____

Prenatal Vitamin Check: Other medicine:

Day of Cycle:	Date:

What's going on in my cycle:

Symptoms:

Exercise and Nutrition:

BBT: CM: CO:
Notes:

My thoughts/feelings:

_____

_____

_____

_____

_____

_____

_____

_____

_____

_____

_____

Prenatal Vitamin Check: Other medicine:

Day of Cycle: Date:

What's going on in my cycle:

Symptoms:

Exercise and Nutrition:

BBT: CM: CO:
Notes:

My thoughts/feelings:

_____

_____

_____

_____

_____

_____

_____

_____

_____

_____

Prenatal Vitamin Check: Other medicine:

Day of Cycle:	Date:

What's going on in my cycle:

Symptoms:

Exercise and Nutrition:

BBT: CM: CO:
Notes:

My thoughts/feelings:

_____

_____

_____

_____

_____

_____

_____

_____

_____

_____

_____

Prenatal Vitamin Check: Other medicine:

Day of Cycle: Date:

What's going on in my cycle:

Symptoms:

Exercise and Nutrition:

BBT: CM: CO:
Notes:

My thoughts/feelings:

_____

_____

_____

_____

_____

_____

_____

_____

_____

_____

_____

Prenatal Vitamin Check: Other medicine:

Day of Cycle: Date:

What's going on in my cycle:

Symptoms:

Exercise and Nutrition:

BBT: CM: CO:
Notes:

My thoughts/feelings:

_____

_____

_____

_____

_____

_____

_____

_____

_____

_____

_____

Prenatal Vitamin Check: Other medicine:

Day of Cycle: Date:

What's going on in my cycle:

Symptoms:

Exercise and Nutrition:

BBT: CM: CO:

Notes:

My thoughts/feelings:

_____

_____

_____

_____

_____

_____

_____

_____

_____

_____

_____

Prenatal Vitamin Check: Other medicine:

Day of Cycle:	Date:

What's going on in my cycle:

Symptoms:

Exercise and Nutrition:

BBT: CM: CO:
Notes:

My thoughts/feelings:

_____

_____

_____

_____

_____

_____

_____

_____

_____

_____

Prenatal Vitamin Check: Other medicine:

Day of Cycle: Date:

What's going on in my cycle:

Symptoms:

Exercise and Nutrition:

BBT: CM: CO:
Notes:

My thoughts/feelings:

_____

_____

_____

_____

_____

_____

_____

_____

_____

_____

_____

Prenatal Vitamin Check: Other medicine:

Day of Cycle: Date:

What's going on in my cycle:

Symptoms:

Exercise and Nutrition:

BBT: CM: CO:
Notes:

My thoughts/feelings:

_____

_____

_____

_____

_____

_____

_____

_____

_____

_____

Prenatal Vitamin Check: Other medicine:

Day of Cycle:	Date:

What's going on in my cycle:

Symptoms:

Exercise and Nutrition:

BBT: CM: CO:

Notes:

My thoughts/feelings:

_____

_____

_____

_____

_____

_____

_____

_____

_____

_____

Prenatal Vitamin Check: Other medicine:

Day of Cycle: Date:

What's going on in my cycle:

Symptoms:

Exercise and Nutrition:

BBT: CM: CO:
Notes:

My thoughts/feelings:

_____

_____

_____

_____

_____

_____

_____

_____

_____

_____

_____

Prenatal Vitamin Check: Other medicine:

Day of Cycle: Date:

What's going on in my cycle:

Symptoms:

Exercise and Nutrition:

BBT: CM: CO:
Notes:

My thoughts/feelings:

_____

_____

_____

_____

_____

_____

_____

_____

_____

_____

Prenatal Vitamin Check: Other medicine:

Day of Cycle:	Date:

What's going on in my cycle:

Symptoms:

Exercise and Nutrition:

BBT:	CM:	CO:

Notes:

My thoughts/feelings:

_____

_____

_____

_____

_____

_____

_____

_____

_____

_____

_____

Prenatal Vitamin Check:	Other medicine:

Day of Cycle: Date:

What's going on in my cycle:

Symptoms:

Exercise and Nutrition:

BBT: CM: CO:
Notes:

My thoughts/feelings:

_____

_____

_____

_____

_____

_____

_____

_____

_____

_____

_____

Prenatal Vitamin Check: Other medicine:

Day of Cycle: Date:

What's going on in my cycle:

Symptoms:

Exercise and Nutrition:

BBT: CM: CO:
Notes:

My thoughts/feelings:

_____

_____

_____

_____

_____

_____

_____

_____

_____

_____

Prenatal Vitamin Check: Other medicine:

Day of Cycle:	Date:

What's going on in my cycle:

Symptoms:

Exercise and Nutrition:

BBT:	CM:	CO:

Notes:

My thoughts/feelings:

_____

_____

_____

_____

_____

_____

_____

_____

_____

_____

Prenatal Vitamin Check:	Other medicine:

Day of Cycle:	Date:

What's going on in my cycle:

Symptoms:

Exercise and Nutrition:

BBT:　　　　　　CM:　　　　　　　CO:
Notes:

My thoughts/feelings:

_____

_____

_____

_____

_____

_____

_____

_____

_____

_____

_____

Prenatal Vitamin Check:　　　　　　Other medicine:

Day of Cycle: Date:

What's going on in my cycle:

Symptoms:

Exercise and Nutrition:

BBT: CM: CO:
Notes:

My thoughts/feelings:

_____

_____

_____

_____

_____

_____

_____

_____

_____

_____

Prenatal Vitamin Check: Other medicine:

Day of Cycle:	Date:

What's going on in my cycle:

Symptoms:

Exercise and Nutrition:

BBT: CM: CO:
Notes:

My thoughts/feelings:

_____

_____

_____

_____

_____

_____

_____

_____

_____

_____

_____

Prenatal Vitamin Check: Other medicine:

Day of Cycle: Date:

What's going on in my cycle:

Symptoms:

Exercise and Nutrition:

BBT: CM: CO:
Notes:

My thoughts/feelings:

_____

_____

_____

_____

_____

_____

_____

_____

_____

_____

_____

Prenatal Vitamin Check: Other medicine:

Day of Cycle: Date:

What's going on in my cycle:

Symptoms:

Exercise and Nutrition:

BBT: CM: CO:

Notes:

My thoughts/feelings:

_____

_____

_____

_____

_____

_____

_____

_____

_____

_____

Prenatal Vitamin Check: Other medicine:

Day of Cycle:	Date:

What's going on in my cycle:

Symptoms:

Exercise and Nutrition:

BBT: CM: CO:
Notes:

My thoughts/feelings:

_____

_____

_____

_____

_____

_____

_____

_____

_____

_____

Prenatal Vitamin Check:	Other medicine:

Day of Cycle: Date:

What's going on in my cycle:

Symptoms:

Exercise and Nutrition:

BBT: CM: CO:
Notes:

My thoughts/feelings:

_____

_____

_____

_____

_____

_____

_____

_____

_____

_____

Prenatal Vitamin Check: Other medicine:

Day of Cycle: Date:

What's going on in my cycle:

Symptoms:

Exercise and Nutrition:

BBT: CM: CO:
Notes:

My thoughts/feelings:

_____

_____

_____

_____

_____

_____

_____

_____

_____

_____

_____

Prenatal Vitamin Check: Other medicine:

Day of Cycle:	Date:

What's going on in my cycle:

Symptoms:

Exercise and Nutrition:

BBT: CM: CO:
Notes:

My thoughts/feelings:

_____

_____

_____

_____

_____

_____

_____

_____

_____

_____

Prenatal Vitamin Check: Other medicine:

Day of Cycle: Date:

What's going on in my cycle:

Symptoms:

Exercise and Nutrition:

BBT: CM: CO:

Notes:

My thoughts/feelings:

_____

_____

_____

_____

_____

_____

_____

_____

_____

_____

Prenatal Vitamin Check: Other medicine:

Day of Cycle: Date:

What's going on in my cycle:

Symptoms:

Exercise and Nutrition:

BBT: CM: CO:

Notes:

My thoughts/feelings:

_____

_____

_____

_____

_____

_____

_____

_____

_____

_____

_____

Prenatal Vitamin Check: Other medicine:

Day of Cycle: Date:

What's going on in my cycle:

Symptoms:

Exercise and Nutrition:

BBT: CM: CO:
Notes:

My thoughts/feelings:

_____

_____

_____

_____

_____

_____

_____

_____

_____

_____

Prenatal Vitamin Check: Other medicine:

Day of Cycle:	Date:

What's going on in my cycle:

Symptoms:

Exercise and Nutrition:

BBT: CM: CO:

Notes:

My thoughts/feelings:

_____

_____

_____

_____

_____

_____

_____

_____

_____

_____

Prenatal Vitamin Check: Other medicine:

Day of Cycle: Date:

What's going on in my cycle:

Symptoms:

Exercise and Nutrition:

BBT: CM: CO:
Notes:

My thoughts/feelings:

_____

_____

_____

_____

_____

_____

_____

_____

_____

_____

_____

Prenatal Vitamin Check: Other medicine:

Day of Cycle: Date:

What's going on in my cycle:

Symptoms:

Exercise and Nutrition:

BBT: CM: CO:
Notes:

My thoughts/feelings:

_____

_____

_____

_____

_____

_____

_____

_____

_____

_____

_____

Prenatal Vitamin Check: Other medicine:

Day of Cycle:	Date:

What's going on in my cycle:

Symptoms:

Exercise and Nutrition:

BBT: CM: CO:
Notes:

My thoughts/feelings:

_____

_____

_____

_____

_____

_____

_____

_____

_____

_____

Prenatal Vitamin Check: Other medicine:

Day of Cycle: Date:

What's going on in my cycle:

Symptoms:

Exercise and Nutrition:

BBT: CM: CO:
Notes:

My thoughts/feelings:

_____

_____

_____

_____

_____

_____

_____

_____

_____

_____

Prenatal Vitamin Check: Other medicine:

Day of Cycle:	Date:

What's going on in my cycle:

Symptoms:

Exercise and Nutrition:

BBT:	CM:	CO:

Notes:

My thoughts/feelings:

_____

_____

_____

_____

_____

_____

_____

_____

_____

_____

Prenatal Vitamin Check:	Other medicine:

Day of Cycle: Date:

What's going on in my cycle:

Symptoms:

Exercise and Nutrition:

BBT: CM: CO:
Notes:

My thoughts/feelings:

_____

_____

_____

_____

_____

_____

_____

_____

_____

_____

Prenatal Vitamin Check: Other medicine:

Day of Cycle: Date:

What's going on in my cycle:

Symptoms:

Exercise and Nutrition:

BBT: CM: CO:
Notes:

My thoughts/feelings:

_____

_____

_____

_____

_____

_____

_____

_____

_____

_____

_____

Prenatal Vitamin Check: Other medicine:

Day of Cycle:	Date:

What's going on in my cycle:

Symptoms:

Exercise and Nutrition:

BBT: CM: CO:
Notes:

My thoughts/feelings:

_____

_____

_____

_____

_____

_____

_____

_____

_____

_____

_____

Prenatal Vitamin Check: Other medicine:

Day of Cycle: Date:

What's going on in my cycle:

Symptoms:

Exercise and Nutrition:

BBT: CM: CO:
Notes:

My thoughts/feelings:

_____

_____

_____

_____

_____

_____

_____

_____

_____

_____

Prenatal Vitamin Check: Other medicine:

Day of Cycle: Date:

What's going on in my cycle:

Symptoms:

Exercise and Nutrition:

BBT: CM: CO:
Notes:

My thoughts/feelings:

_____

_____

_____

_____

_____

_____

_____

_____

_____

_____

_____

Prenatal Vitamin Check: Other medicine:

Day of Cycle:	Date:

What's going on in my cycle:

Symptoms:

Exercise and Nutrition:

BBT: CM: CO:
Notes:

My thoughts/feelings:

_____

_____

_____

_____

_____

_____

_____

_____

_____

_____

Prenatal Vitamin Check: Other medicine:

Day of Cycle:	Date:

What's going on in my cycle:

Symptoms:

Exercise and Nutrition:

BBT: CM: CO:
Notes:

My thoughts/feelings:

_____

_____

_____

_____

_____

_____

_____

_____

_____

_____

Prenatal Vitamin Check: Other medicine:

Day of Cycle: Date:

What's going on in my cycle:

Symptoms:

Exercise and Nutrition:

BBT: CM: CO:
Notes:

My thoughts/feelings:

_____

_____

_____

_____

_____

_____

_____

_____

_____

_____

_____

Prenatal Vitamin Check: Other medicine:

Day of Cycle: Date:

What's going on in my cycle:

Symptoms:

Exercise and Nutrition:

BBT: CM: CO:

Notes:

My thoughts/feelings:

_____

_____

_____

_____

_____

_____

_____

_____

_____

_____

Prenatal Vitamin Check: Other medicine:

Day of Cycle: Date:

What's going on in my cycle:

Symptoms:

Exercise and Nutrition:

BBT: CM: CO:
Notes:

My thoughts/feelings:

_____

_____

_____

_____

_____

_____

_____

_____

_____

_____

_____

Prenatal Vitamin Check: Other medicine:

Day of Cycle:	Date:

What's going on in my cycle:

Symptoms:

Exercise and Nutrition:

BBT: CM: CO:
Notes:

My thoughts/feelings:

_____

_____

_____

_____

_____

_____

_____

_____

_____

_____

_____

Prenatal Vitamin Check: Other medicine:

Day of Cycle: Date:

What's going on in my cycle:

Symptoms:

Exercise and Nutrition:

BBT: CM: CO:

Notes:

My thoughts/feelings:

_____

_____

_____

_____

_____

_____

_____

_____

_____

_____

Prenatal Vitamin Check: Other medicine:

Day of Cycle: Date:

What's going on in my cycle:

Symptoms:

Exercise and Nutrition:

BBT: CM: CO:

Notes:

My thoughts/feelings:

_____

_____

_____

_____

_____

_____

_____

_____

_____

_____

Prenatal Vitamin Check: Other medicine:

Day of Cycle: Date:

What's going on in my cycle:

Symptoms:

Exercise and Nutrition:

BBT: CM: CO:
Notes:

My thoughts/feelings:

_____

_____

_____

_____

_____

_____

_____

_____

_____

_____

_____

Prenatal Vitamin Check: Other medicine:

Day of Cycle:	Date:

What's going on in my cycle:

Symptoms:

Exercise and Nutrition:

BBT:　　　　　　CM:　　　　　　CO:

Notes:

My thoughts/feelings:

_____

_____

_____

_____

_____

_____

_____

_____

_____

_____

Prenatal Vitamin Check:　　　　　Other medicine:

Day of Cycle: Date:

What's going on in my cycle:

Symptoms:

Exercise and Nutrition:

BBT: CM: CO:

Notes:

My thoughts/feelings:

_____

_____

_____

_____

_____

_____

_____

_____

_____

Prenatal Vitamin Check: Other medicine:

Day of Cycle: Date:

What's going on in my cycle:

Symptoms:

Exercise and Nutrition:

BBT: CM: CO:
Notes:

My thoughts/feelings:

_____

_____

_____

_____

_____

_____

_____

_____

_____

_____

_____

Prenatal Vitamin Check: Other medicine:

Day of Cycle: Date:

What's going on in my cycle:

Symptoms:

Exercise and Nutrition:

BBT: CM: CO:

Notes:

My thoughts/feelings:

_____

_____

_____

_____

_____

_____

_____

_____

_____

_____

_____

Prenatal Vitamin Check: Other medicine:

Day of Cycle:	Date:

What's going on in my cycle:

Symptoms:

Exercise and Nutrition:

BBT: CM: CO:
Notes:

My thoughts/feelings:

_____

_____

_____

_____

_____

_____

_____

_____

_____

_____

_____

Prenatal Vitamin Check: Other medicine:

Day of Cycle:	Date:

What's going on in my cycle:

Symptoms:

Exercise and Nutrition:

BBT: CM: CO:

Notes:

My thoughts/feelings:

_____

_____

_____

_____

_____

_____

_____

_____

_____

_____

Prenatal Vitamin Check: Other medicine:

Day of Cycle:	Date:

What's going on in my cycle:

Symptoms:

Exercise and Nutrition:

BBT: CM: CO:
Notes:

My thoughts/feelings:

_____

_____

_____

_____

_____

_____

_____

_____

_____

_____

_____

Prenatal Vitamin Check: Other medicine:

Day of Cycle:	Date:

What's going on in my cycle:

Symptoms:

Exercise and Nutrition:

BBT: CM: CO:

Notes:

My thoughts/feelings:

_____

_____

_____

_____

_____

_____

_____

_____

_____

_____

_____

Prenatal Vitamin Check: Other medicine:

Day of Cycle: Date:

What's going on in my cycle:

Symptoms:

Exercise and Nutrition:

BBT: CM: CO:

Notes:

My thoughts/feelings:

_____

_____

_____

_____

_____

_____

_____

_____

_____

_____

Prenatal Vitamin Check: Other medicine:

www.ingramcontent.com/pod-product-compliance
Lightning Source LLC
Chambersburg PA
CBHW051345280526
45784CB00007B/2817